I0706558

<u>KNOW THE 18 FOODS THAT WILL KEEP YOU FRESH THROUGHOUT THE DAY</u>

Raisins

 Soak raisins overnight in water and eat them with water the next morning. These will keep your body energized throughout the day. As a result, you will also be fresh.

Dal

Dal also plays an effective role in keeping you fresh throughout the day. Eating half-boiled dal during breakfast every morning helps to store energy in the body. This increases people's motivation to work. Moreover, it can be eaten with lunch.

The Egg

Eggs are the most efficient food for energy storage. You can eat eggs every day for breakfast or with lunch. It will keep your body fresh and active by saving your body energy.

Lemon

Lemon is very effective in storing energy in the body. In summer you can mix lemon juice with sugar, water and mint to make syrup and eat it. This drink helps to keep the body fresh.

Sweet Potato

 Sweet potatoes contain carbohydrates; which fulfills the energy needs of the body. It lowers blood sugar levels and helps keep you energized throughout the day.

Garlic

 Eating a little garlic with food every day is good for health. This food purifies the blood and brightens the skin.

Onion

Eating 3-4 small raw onions in lunch every day keeps the body fresh. It controls diabetes by lowering blood sugar levels and removes excess fat.

Cumin

 Boiling cumin seeds and drinking water improves digestion. It is also good food for digestive system.

Sugar

Palm sugar is more effective than cane sugar in keeping the body fresh. Because it contains less calories. So eat this food regularly to stay fresh throughout the day.

Soup

After the operation, if you have a cold or body ache, eating the soup will help you recover quickly. The ginger and chilies in the chicken soup work to solve these problems quickly.

Jau

Jau plays an effective role in solving stomach pain or digestive problems. Jau is made with a mixture of rice, garlic and onion; Which saves the energy needed to solve the problem.

Olive Oil

Cooking with olive oil does not accumulate fat in the body. It increases blood flow in the body. As a result, the body remains fresh.

Mushroom

Mushroom soup can be consumed as an alternative to milk tea and coffee. It also plays an effective role in keeping the body fresh.

Banana

Banana works in energy storage. Eating banana before going to bed at night keeps energy in the body. As a result, the body remains fresh the next day.

Honey

Honey is a source of energy. Daily consumption of honey mixed with hot lemon juice makes the body fresh and more vibrant.

<u>Important topic note please</u>

<u>**EXERCISE TO KEEP THE BODY HEALTHY**</u>

Drink water and kushal on an empty stomach after waking up

Good health

Be well, be

Take care of the body, choose the right food, diagnose the cause of the disease and how to prevent it, without giving medicine.

Thomas Alva Edison, American inventor
Although it is possible to implement what Edison predicted today, we are still not aware enough about body care, diet and disease prevention. So this is a small attempt to write something based on the advice of various humanitarian doctors and researchers.

1. Proper exercise and diet and a cheerful mind are the keys to staying healthy. In fact, we have so much anxiety or tension in our lives that we cannot be happy. But as the saying goes, the grave is filled with tension more than the grave is filled with cancer. So if you want to live well, you have to keep your mind cheerful. There is no substitute for good thoughts and good deeds. Along with that you have to involve yourself with some creative work.

2. Exercise should be started from the age of four. There are many types of exercise. Such as walking, swimming and running-jumping, exercise by running a bicycle or other equipment and lifting something heavy, exercise by massaging different parts of the body and yoga exercise by keeping the body fixed in a special posture. All exercise is beneficial. However, it is better to choose exercise considering age, physical positional needs, environmental benefits, time constraints and mental inclinations. But there are some exercises that can be done by anyone unless they are completely bedridden or immobile. Emphasis is placed on them in this article.

3. Walk briskly for 45 minutes every day. If not at once, several times. In this, all the body parts are flexible and the brain gets a lot of oxygen, anxiety is reduced. Walking also prevents menopausal osteoporosis and other complications in women.

4. Limb movements and massaging are good exercises. Because blood circulation is easy in it, fat cannot accumulate. Here are mentioned massages in some important parts of the body by which both the proximal and distal organs are benefited.

A) Whenever possible, massaging the whole head keeps the brain and nerve center healthy because the blood circulates well in the head and hair does not fall or grow easily.

B) Daily 10 minutes of massaging the wet forehead by turning the hands keeps the pituitary gland responsible for physical growth fresh.

C) Massaging the front and back of the ear and twisting the ear along with the earlobe is good for the stomach.

D) If the tip of the nose is rotated with the palm of the hand, the kidneys are strong.

E) Neck is the first victim of any stress of body and mind. So massaging the neck and tilting the head up and down and around keeps the neck flexible.

F) Thyroid and tonsil glands are good if massaged on both sides of the neck under the jaw.

G) Hands are very mobile by applying light pressure on elbow joint and massaging normally between elbow and wrist.

H) Massaging around the navel reduces anxiety and does not easily cause bowel disturbances if done lying down.

5. Lying down with two hands on the stomach and inhaling deeply through the nose and exhaling slowly through the mouth increases lung power and 20 minutes a day leads to good sleep. Continuously contracting and releasing the anus for as long as possible is a very good exercise to increase the overall strength of the body and retain youth.

6. A large portion of the nervous system terminates in the palms of the hands and soles of the feet. For this, clapping hands removes cataracts, lowers high blood pressure and improves memory. Rubbing the soles of the feet with something rough, such as a dhundul or a plastic brush, for a total of 20 minutes a day stimulates all the body parts, keeps them fresh and heals them slowly even if they are sick. It is particularly beneficial in preventing insomnia, heart disease and stroke, and during pregnancy in women. After rubbing the soles of the feet, move the fingers up and down.

7. Splash water 25 times in the eyes while washing the face. Inhale and exhale as much water as possible through the nose. It will not cause cold and cough easily. In addition, it is very beneficial in headache, sinusitis and migraine.

8. The practice of yoga invented in our subcontinent is now popular all over the world, but many of us are ignorant about it. However, many well-written books on yoga exercises are available these days. Read these and if possible get a proper idea from an expert. The main feature of this exercise is various postures called asanas. Each asana puts pressure on the body in one way which benefits each part of the body. After staying in these asanas for some time, one has to rest in a special asana called Shavasana.

9. Keeping the mind free from worries, one has to lie down without a pillow and spread his arms and legs. When you wake up in the morning, take a short nap without jumping out of bed. It increases strength and confidence. Daily Shavasana for half an hour keeps the spine healthy, can withstand a lot of work and stress and removes any pain and hidden problems in the body. Note that most of the blood is produced from the bone marrow of the spine and ribs.

10. In the morning, before breakfast, do two more yoga poses: Pawanmuktasana and Bhujangasana. Air accumulated in the stomach during digestion at night is responsible for one-third of all diseases. The upper two asanas clear the stomach and increase digestion. Pawanmuktasana is also beneficial for asthma, back and waist pain and polyuria or diabetes patients. Bhujangasana also relieves all types of back and waist pain, high blood pressure and gynecological disorders. No other yogasana can be done after eating except Vajrasana. Vajrasana aids in digestion and sleep and strengthens the body from the waist to the feet.

11. Now on the subject of food (this is a very touchy subject, because many of us live to eat rather than eat to live).

A) Nutritionists say, "You are what you eat." A major reason for the many complex diseases that have overtaken us today is that the original purity of food has been lost in this era of artificial fertilizers and pesticides. On top of that there are various processed, adulterated and chemically preserved foods which can in no way be equal to pure and fresh foods. Food stored in the refrigerator for a long time is also harmful. But healthy cells need pure blood which is made only from pure and fresh food.

B) A quality component in food is fiber which keeps the intestinal tract clean thus preventing cancer. Wheat flour has fiber, flour does not. Flour is a processed dead food that contributes to constipation and cancer. Another such processed food is sugar, which causes many serious diseases, increases blood density and even erodes bones. So it is better to avoid food made of flour and sugar completely. Also oil, salt and spices should be used in nominal quantity.

C) Consume 40% of your daily diet with white vegetables, 15% of meat and 45% of vegetables and fruits. But don't eat fruits with white foods like rice, bread, potatoes etc.; Eat at least half an hour apart. It is also not good to eat non-vegetarian food such as fish, meat, eggs with white sugar. Vegetables are the only food that can be eaten with both meat and protein. Eat at least half a kg of vegetables a day. Start your morning with plenty of raw papaya and fruit. It will be good for the liver. Sprouted wheat, chickpeas, mung beans, chickpeas etc. and foods made from flour and barley are good for breakfast. Vegetables, beans and cabbages should be eaten during the day as they produce flatulence in the stomach at night.

D) Pulses are excellent as a source of meat. Especially mung, lentil and muscalli. Apart from that, chickpeas and sprouted chickpeas fulfill the deficiency of non-vegetables in the human body of all ages and are good for polyuria. Boiled soybeans contain substances that are beneficial in polyuria and protect the prostate gland in men and the uterus in women. For animal meats, fish, chicken and egg whites are good. Red meat i.e. beef is delicious but it is a source of many serious diseases due to harmful fats.

E) After drinking at least 600 grams of water before brushing teeth in the morning, stop drinking for 45 minutes. It cleanses the colon and cures many complex diseases including acidity. Drink 8/10 glasses of water a day. Girls should never drink water standing up, it damages the uterus. Light tea without milk is good as a healthy drink. Bottled water is also good, but not more than one a day. Drink lemon water mixed with honey or a little jaggery to boost your energy in summer and stay away from all soft drinks. Because these sherbets, marketed with only profit-making formulas and filled with attractive bottles shown in shiny advertisements, are full of sugar and deliciousness, they are the cause of many major diseases, including diabetes. (With the addition of fast food, the basis for fast death has been created.)

F) Quantity and timing of intake are also important. Never eat full. It should be eaten at the same time every day. It is better to have dinner by eight o'clock. Because the digestive power decreases from the afternoon.

12. A short list of disease-preventing foods and drinks: Barley is beneficial in polyuria, lowers cholesterol and keeps the skin and colon healthy. Gamankur is anti-cancer. Daily some amount of sour curd and in the morning a glass of green vegetable juice (cabbage, kalmi, thankuni, lettuce, telakucha, patharkuchi etc.) made by mixing water, if possible mix with honey, dry ginger and triphala i.e. dry amlaki, haritaki and bahera powder. It keeps the body fresh.
Similarly, it is good to drink raw papaya, vegetables like carrot and gourd and juice of fruits like kamaranga and grapefruit. By slicing raw bel and drying it in the sun, soaking or boiling bel pods and eating them regularly with water can cure many old stomach ailments, such as indigestion and dysentery. Kalmi leaves keep the skin healthy and heals wounds. Raw greens build and purify the blood. Thankuni leaves are good for stomach, eyes and hair. Mint leaves are good for lungs, heart and stomach. Ginger relieves rheumatism and headaches and improves digestion.

Amalki is the best source of Vitamin C. Sesame retains youth. Raw turmeric is a good blood purifier. Kaljira has been called a medicine for thousands of diseases since ancient times. Spirulina replenishes body waste and is beneficial in many diseases including high blood pressure and diabetes. Garlic-boiled water prevents colds and coughs.

13. Many diseases are caused by oral hygiene. So brush your teeth before going to bed at night and shake off all the worries of your mind by doing shavasan before sleeping on a fairly firm bed.

14. What has been said in so few words is a small part of the vast body of knowledge related to health. But if you want to know more about this in a short and easy way to stay healthy through self-medication, you can read Chinmoy Sengupta's "Drug-Free Disease Cure/Preticin Program" and Devendra Vora's "Your Health in Your Hands/Acupressure and Other Natural Treatments".

Health is the root of all happiness
"Health is the root of all happiness" - you must have heard it from your elders. In fact, apart from well-being, another meaning of health is happiness. When there is disease, happiness goes away, so disease is called disease.
Knowing and practicing how to avoid illness, or how to get well and stay well, is very important. Especially at a young age like you.

Then you will not get sick easily and you will be able to live a long life in a healthy body. Before getting to know health rules well, remember one thing that body and mind are connected together. So both should be given importance.
 If you compare the body with a machine, you will see that just as the machine needs oil, gas or electricity, the body also needs food, drink and air. As long as the air is unpolluted, there's a lot to think about when it comes to food and drink.

First thing, we eat to live or live to eat? Gluttons or 'eaters' may believe that we should live to eat, but most people think we eat to live. That is the truth. Eating habits are taking good quality food and drink in right amount at right time. Stomach is never overfilled, it causes digestive disturbances. It should be eaten at the same time every day. It is better to have dinner by eight o'clock, because digestion starts to slow down in the afternoon.

Now let's see what to eat. Foods that are easily digestible should be eaten at all times. As it does not put too much pressure on the digestive system, the stomach does not get upset and the nutrients from the food are well added to the body.

Foods with excess oil, fat, salt and spices and fried foods should not be eaten at all. It also wastes things and health.

A beneficial component of food is fiber which keeps the bowels clean and prevents stomach cancer easily. Cancer is a very serious disease. If the food is rubbed or mixed with chemicals to make it white, smooth and delicate, the fiber will disappear. Such food is called dead food. Flour and white sugar are dead foods. It is better not to eat food made with them. Because just as flour can cause cancer, sugar can erode our bones.

But it's just that sweet things are fun to eat. So if you want to eat something sweet, you can look for a source other than sugar. For example, jaggery or honey can be eaten in small quantities. Sweet fruits are best. Sugary drinks are also bad. Especially soft drinks. Also, the habit of eating various delicious foods made of flour, oil, butter, etc., such as parathas, breads, biscuits, chips, noodles, semai, cakes, pastries, patties, chanachurs, burgers and various 'fast food' can lead to serious diseases, such as heart disease, high blood pressure. causing high blood pressure, polyuria or diabetes. The rate of polyuria among young people in Asia has increased and continues to increase due to this alone.

People are slaves to habits. So you should try to give up eating tasty but bad food and eat good food even if it tastes a little less at first. If you don't have a habit of eating junk food, you don't have to give up that habit with difficulty. This also applies to smoking and drug addiction.

As a percentage, 40 percent of the food should be white i.e. rice-bread, 15 percent non-vegetarian i.e. fish-meat-egg-dal and the remaining 45 percent vegetables-vegetables-fruits. Because beef and khasi meat contains fat, it is dangerous and eating too much can cause serious diseases. It is good to eat at least half a kg of vegetables a day. There should be quite a bit of raw papaya for breakfast. And there must be any kind of fruit. Five kinds of fruits and six kinds of vegetables should be eaten every day.

Vegetables can be eaten in three meals. However, eating vegetables such as greens, beans and cabbage at night accumulates gas in the stomach. Morning is the most important time of the day to eat. Noon is less important than morning and night is less important than noon. Many people get sick by eating more at noon than at breakfast and at night than at noon without knowing it.

Fresh food produces pure blood and pure blood keeps the cells of the body healthy. For this you should not eat solid food. If food is kept in the fridge for too long, its quality and taste will be lost. 2 to 3 liters of water should be consumed a day to replenish the majority of body water. Among them, after drinking 600 grams (2 to 3 glasses) of water on an empty stomach in the morning, after stopping drinking for 45 minutes, bowel movements are easy and many complex diseases including acidity are cured. Bottled water is also good, but not more than one a day. Light tea without milk and sugar is beneficial.

 Apart from being selective in food and drink intake, proper exercise is needed to keep the body and mind active. Exercise is more important in children because it develops their body structure and personality. There are many methods of exercise. Walking, running, jumping and various games based on these and swimming are forms of exercise. Another type of exercise is done with the help of bicycles or various equipment.

There is another type of exercise that doesn't require running or equipment, but is very beneficial. Its name is yoga exercise. This exercise is done by alternately putting pressure on different parts of the body and relaxing it. There are many books about its rules, some even teach this exercise. You read books and learn yoga exercises from someone if you have a chance.

There is no harm without gain if you continue with other exercises. For example, walking. Walking briskly for at least half an hour every day reduces anxiety or tension as the body is flexible and a lot of oxygen enters the brain.

 Different postures in yoga exercises are called asanas. Here are four essential asanas that people of all ages should do.

Shavasana The first is Shavasana.

This name refers to lying in an inanimate posture like a corpse. This name is given to the hands and feet without a pillow in this seat. In this seat, without a pillow, you have to lie down with your arms and legs spread out and your mind free from worries. It can be done at any time and half an hour daily is good for the spine. Most of the blood is produced from the bone marrow of the spine and ribs.

Apart from that, doing this asana can withstand a lot of work and mental stress, remembers reading and removes any pain and hidden problems in the body. Doing this for a while without jumping out of bed in the morning increases energy and confidence. But the bed should not be so soft that the spine bends when sleeping.

The second and third seats are Pavanmuktasana and Bhujangasana.

Both of these can be done before breakfast or in the evening. Air that accumulates in the stomach during digestion is responsible for three-fourths of all diseases. By doing these two asanas, the stomach becomes free of air and improves digestion. Apart from that Pawanmuktasana is beneficial in polyuria and asthma. Bhujangasana relieves all types of back and waist pain, high blood pressure and feminine ailments.

The fourth asana is Vajrasana, which is performed immediately after eating. It helps in digestion and sleep and keeps the spine healthy. Despite this, various yogasanas or other exercises can be done according to the different needs of the body.
 The descriptions of the above three asanas except Shavasana are briefly given below.

Pawanmuktasana: Lying straight, first fold the right leg from the knee and place it on the stomach and chest and hold it with both hands. Keeping breathing normal, count from ten to thirty in your mind. Then lower the right leg and rest. Do the seat twice.

Pawanmuktasana (a)
Pawanmuktasana (b)
It will be called once when the number is counted by pressing the left foot and then both feet. Shavasana should be done three times in a row with equal time rest.

Bhujangasana: Lie down with both legs straight. Place the palms of both hands on the floor next to the ribs. Now keep the feet on the floor from the waist and lift the head as far as possible by resting on the palms of the hands. Now bend your head back as far as you can and look up. Stay in this position for 25-30 seconds with normal breathing. Then slowly lower your head and chest and lie down and rest Bhujangasana

Vajrasana: Bend your knees and fold your legs behind you and sit with your head straight in a prayer posture. Place your palms on both knees. The butt will be on the ankle. The first few days may be a little difficult. So sit in that position as long as you can. If you cannot stay for a long time at a time, do the asana thrice keeping the breath normal and rest in shavasana.

Vajrasana
Nerves keep the mind in touch with the body. All the nerves together form the nervous system, a large portion of which terminates in the soles of the feet. For that reason, if you rub the soles of your feet with something rough, such as dhundul bark or a plastic brush, the body stays refreshed and the sick body recovers slowly. So every day whenever possible rub the bottom of each foot for at least ten minutes and pull the fingers up and down.

 While washing the face, splash water several times in the eyes. If you draw water through your nose as much as possible and release it, you will not get cold or headache easily.

 Must brush your teeth before going to bed at night, because many diseases are caused by oral hygiene. Apart from that, whenever you eat something or drink something other than water, rinsing well with water will keep your teeth healthy. And you know, it is wise to understand the status of teeth to have teeth!

<u>Important topic note please</u>

<u>A QUICK WAY TO INCREASE BODY ENERGY</u>

Do you feel tired all the time? Do you always fall asleep no matter what? Sometimes the body feels tired due to lack of energy. Some energy boosting tips are given which if followed you will see the problem reduced a lot.

Don't Skip Breakfast : Breakfast is the first meal of the day. So it determines the energy level of your body throughout the day. Therefore, if you do not have breakfast, the body does not store new energy. As a result, your body's energy gradually decreases as time goes by. So have breakfast in the morning with foods that are rich in carbohydrates and proteins.
 Balanced diet: Don't skip lunch or any other meal of the day just because you have a good breakfast. Eat plenty of fruits every day in addition to protein and carbohydrate-rich foods. Also include energy boosting foods such as eggs, oats or nuts in the diet.

Exercise: No matter how much you eat the right food, if you don't exercise properly, there will be no benefit. Be it jogging in the morning or an evening walk in the evening, any exercise is very useful for the body.
Drink plenty of water: Sometimes drinking less water can leave you feeling drained and dizzy. Drink at least 7 to 8 glasses of water a day.
 Don't get stressed out at all: Being stressed can quickly lead to low energy levels. During this time, try deep breathing, listen to good music or watch a good movie or reduce stress with meditation.

Change bad habits: After consumption of alcohol or cigarettes, the energy level increases for a while but in the long run it is harmful. So avoid these two.

Be around smiling and happy people: It has been found that negative emotions such as anger, jealousy, frustration increase stress and decrease energy. So try to be among smiling happy people as much as you can.

<u>Important topic note please</u>

<u>TECHNIQUES TO INCREASE BODY STRENGTH</u>

Here is a list of 19 foods that increase physical strength based on health magazine.

This food list is:
Seafood, green peppers, green fruits like avocados or pears, chocolate, bananas, honey, coffee, watermelon, pine nuts, cherries, sweet pumpkin seeds, green leafy vegetables, olive oil, figs, strawberries, artichokes, raisins and currants. . According to experts, amino acids in seafood, endorphins in chili peppers, vitamin C in avocados, dopamine in dark chocolate, bromoline in bananas, boron in honey, mood enhancers in coffee, lycopene in watermelon, zinc in pine nuts, mono and polyunsaturated fats in olive oil, magnesium in currants are body energy sources. effective in growth.

These ingredients have many benefits including increasing the production of the hormone testosterone, which is necessary for increasing the strength of the male body, improving the body's immune system and improving the mood. As a result, eating these food ingredients increases the strength of the body and can stay well without medicine

Does the strength increase only by increasing the weight of the set? This is a method of increasing energy that everyone knows. Today we will talk about some other techniques that will help you increase your strength very quickly. These are just a few techniques you can apply during any workout.

Increase exercise range
If we want to train ourselves a little harder, we usually complete the set by increasing the weight. It's definitely good. It is also possible to put different pressures on the muscles by making some small changes in the exercise. For example, keeping the chest as close to the ground as possible while doing pushups, keeping the hips high, and keeping the elbows straight while lifting.

Increase exercise range
If we want to train ourselves a little harder, we usually complete the set by increasing the weight. It's definitely good. It is also possible to put different pressures on the muscles by making some small changes in the exercise. For example, keeping the chest as close to the ground as possible while doing pushups, keeping the hips high, and keeping the elbows straight while lifting.

Do something hard
Bring variation to exercise. Strain specific muscles. Let's say the single leg squat is more difficult than the regular squat. It puts your entire body weight on one leg. Moreover, you have to keep an eye on maintaining the balance of the body. All in all a tough exercise.

Exercise slowly
Will the muscle pressure be
read only if you complete
the set in a hurry? Try to do
the correct reps gradually.
Slow down the exercises
that you used to do in a
hurry. You will notice the
difference immediately.

Know, change
Check out the experienced
bodybuilders. See their
exercise technique, know.
Try to vary your exercise by
comparison. And practice.
Because the more you
practice a thing, the more
you can master it.

Eating a meal in the morning increases the energy in the body many times!
We eat many kinds of food every day to meet the different nutrients of the body but do we all know what kind of food can increase our sex?

Generally, when the balance of vitamins and minerals in food is right, the endocrine system in the body is active.

And it controls the production of estrogen and testosterone in your body.

Estrogen and testosterone are essential for sex drive and performance.

Your diet has a lot to do with whether you're in the mood for sex.

Increases power in the body manifold.

Milk:

These natural foods that are high in animal-fat can improve your sex life. For example, pure milk, milk syrup, butter etc.

Most people want to avoid fatty foods.

But if you want to increase the production of sex hormones in the body, then you need to eat a lot of fat.

But they should all be natural and saturated fats.

<u>Important topic note please</u>

A problem is becoming quite apparent among most men. Impotence in men is increasing day by day. In addition, with the increase in age, the sexual desire of men is gradually decreasing. So it is necessary to be aware before the sexual demand decreases You can know how this demand is gradually declining

Home remedies have come forward to solve this problem in men Home remedies are the way for them to regain their full sex drive Home remedies can be effective in those who have just experienced this problem Some cases can be treated with home remedies but not all home remedies are applicable

Now let's know what materials can be used in daily life in the treatment of the first stage of sexual impotence or what are the benefits of using them-

Garlic:

Garlic is very effective in sexual impotence Garlic is called the 'poor man's penicillin' Because it acts as an antiseptic Which we almost always take as food
 Its use is very effective in bringing back your sexual desire It helps you regain your sex drive if you lose it due to an illness or an accident Garlic is also very effective in cases where a person's sexual desire is too high or excessive, where excessive use can damage the nervous system.

Chew two to three cloves of raw garlic daily It will increase your sex drive if it has decreased Also, mixing wheat bread with garlic increases the sperm production level in your body and helps in healthy sperm production.

Onion:

Onion has long been used as an aphrodisiac
and aphrodisiac But how it works in this
regard is not yet known exactly
 Grind white onion and fry it well in butter
and eat it daily with honey. But remember
one thing, keep your stomach empty for
couple of hours before consuming it In this
way, it is possible to solve the problem of
slipping, premature falling or falling during
sleep by playing it daily

 Also soak the powder of Beuli dal with
black peel in onion juice for seven days and
dry it. Its regular use will maintain your
libido and stamina during sexual
intercourse.

Carrot:

One and a half hundred grams of grated
carrot mixed with one tablespoon of honey
and half-boiled egg for two months can
reduce your physical disability.

<u>FOOD TO INCREASE BODY STRENGTH
WITHOUT DRUGS</u>

Many people ask what kind of food can increase physical strength. Increases blood circulation in the body. Some necessary hormones are produced. The mood is fresh and so on. Those of us who are doctors and who mercilessly prescribe piles of drugs when needed don't always think about alternative treatments. But many people are thinking about exercise and food to increase physical capacity without medicine. Here is a list of 19 foods that increase physical strength based on foreign health magazines. This food list is:

 Seafood, green peppers, pear-like green fruits, chocolate, bananas, honey, coffee, watermelon, pine nuts, cherries, sweet pumpkin seeds, green leafy vegetables, olive oil, figs, strawberries, artichokes, raisins and currants.

According to experts, amino acids in marine fish, endorphins in peppers, vitamin C in pears, dopamine in dark chocolate, bromoline in bananas, boron in honey, mood-enhancing ingredients in coffee, lycopene in watermelon, zinc in pine nuts, mono and polyunsaturated fats in olive oil, magnesium in currants, body energy. effective in growth.

These ingredients have many benefits including increasing the production of the hormone testosterone, which is necessary for increasing the strength of the male body, improving the body's immune system and improving the mood. As a result, eating these food ingredients increases the strength of the body and can stay well without medicine.

<u>Important topic note please</u>

<u>10 FOODS THAT INCREASE
SPERM COUNT</u>

A balanced diet is required for body nutrition. A nutritious diet not only maintains your physical health but also affects your sexual health. Here we will talk about 10 foods that will help in increasing sperm along with providing energy to the body.

1. The Egg

Vitamins present in eggs increase fertility. Antioxidants protect sex cells from becoming dysfunctional.

2. Dark Chocolate

Eating dark chocolate increases sperm count in men. As a result, the sperm count also increases.

3. Tomato

Lycopene levels are very low in people suffering from infertility. Keratonite lycopene helps increase sperm count and activity. Tomatoes are a very good source of these antioxidants.

4. The Carrot

Vitamins present in carrots help to strengthen the nervous system and increase sexual activity in men.

5. Spinach

Spinach, rich in folic acid, helps in increasing the number of sperm and helps it to function well.

6. Walnut

Walnuts increase the volume of semen.
It also helps in sperm production.
Walnuts contain omega-3 fatty acids that
improve blood circulation in men.

7. Currants

Currant contains antioxidants. Which
reduces the amount of sperm growth in
the body reduces the amount of
melondialdehyde in the body. As a
result, sperm potency increases.

8. Garlic

Garlic is rich in vitamin B6 and selenium.
Eating garlic increases libido. Being a
good source of allicin, garlic also
improves blood circulation in the sexual
organs.

9. Oranges

Consuming an orange every day increases the body's immune system. Consuming it daily will improve your sex life. In Ayurveda, orange is said to be a storehouse of virtue.

10. Banana

Banana contains vitamins A, C, B1. Helps in sperm production and increases sexual potency. Bananas contain the enzyme bromelain which helps regulate sex hormones.

<u>FOODS THAT INCREASE SEXUAL ENERGY
IN THE BODY IN A NATURAL WAY</u>

Side-effect medicinal techniques and psychological treatments to enhance libido are now almost obsolete. Nowadays, natural aphrodisiacs or sexual enhancement foods are considered to be more effective in increasing libido. So to stay sexually fit in married life, you need to pay full attention to daily diet. Because for a happy married life, a healthy sex life is needed along with a good understanding between husband and wife.

However, it is often seen that due to sexual problems, there is turmoil in the family, and even divorce. So even if you are careful in advance, you may not face such a situation. You don't need any kind of medicine to increase your sexual power, it is enough to eat nutritious food daily. Keep regular milk, eggs and honey in your food menu and lead a regular life, then you will not suffer from sexual weakness.

Eggs:

Milk is an excellent food to remove sexual weakness and increase sexual arousal. Eat 1 boiled egg every morning, if not at least 5 days a week. This will solve your sexual weakness.

Milk:

A natural diet that is high in animal-fat can improve your sex life. For example, pure milk, milk syrup, butter etc. Most people want to avoid fatty foods. But if you want to increase the production of sex hormones in the body, you need a lot of fatty foods. But all should be natural and saturated fats.

Honey:

Everyone is more or less aware of the healing properties of honey for sexual impotence. So drink 1 glass of hot water mixed with 1 spoon of pure honey at least 3/4 days every week to increase sexual energy.

Garlic:

If you have sexual problems, start eating garlic regularly now. Since time immemorial, the nutritional value of garlic has been widely recognized in both men and women to increase sexual arousal and keep the genitals fully functional. Garlic contains a substance called allicin that increases blood flow to the genitals.

Coffee:

Coffee plays an important role in increasing your sex drive. The caffeine in coffee keeps your sexual mood active.

Jaiphal:

Studies have shown that Jaiphal releases an aphrodisiac compound. In general, this compound stimulates nerve cells and increases blood circulation. As a result, your sex drive increases. You can mix jaiphal with coffee, then it is possible to get the two functions together.

Chocolate:

Chocolate has always been associated with love and sex. It contains phenylethylamine (PEA) and serotonin. These two substances are also present in our brain. They are helpful in increasing sexual arousal and energy levels in the body. Anandamide together with PEA helps to reach orgasm.

Banana:

Banana contains vitamins A, B, C and potassium. Vitamin B and potassium increase the production of semen in the human body. And bananas also contain bromelain. Which is also helpful in increasing the testosterone levels in the body. And above all, bananas are rich in carbohydrates that boost your body's energy. As a result, you will not get tired even if you engage in sexual intercourse for a long time.

Fruits rich in Vitamin C:

If you want to maintain good sexual health, include colorful fruits in your daily diet. Fruits such as grapes, oranges, watermelons, peaches etc. are very beneficial for increasing sexual power. Studies have shown that a man who has at least 200 mg of vitamin C in his daily diet improves the quality of his sperm. Among these fruits, the effect of watermelon is more. Many have compared watermelon to the sex-stimulating drug Viagra.

Beef:

Beef is rich in zinc. So you eat low-fat beef to make your sex life more enjoyable. Like beef shoulder, venison is low in fat and high in zinc. Meat from these areas contains 10 mg of zinc per 100 grams.

Foods that increase energy

People have to be busy with some work all day long. Even in the middle of this busy time they have to sleep. As the saying goes, health is the root of all happiness. Therefore, it is important to be aware in every aspect of life besides sleep to maintain health. There are certain foods that can be consumed regularly to stay fresh throughout the day. At the same time, these foods help to keep the body calm.

<u>Important topic note please</u>

<u>**7 INGREDIENTS TO ENHANCE THE QUALITY OF HERBAL TEA**</u>

Herbal tea is good for your health. And if you can add some extra ingredients to it, it will improve as well as taste.

By adding these ingredients to herbal tea, it is possible to get various herbal properties that are beneficial for health. Seven such elements are described in this text-

1. Lemon

Lemon will increase the taste and smell of herbal tea manifold. This is one way to add vitamin C to tea. And it also works well to remove toxins from the body. Lemon reduces stress. And it also benefits digestion.

2. Ginger

Ginger slices or ginger powder can be used in herbal tea. And it's also very easy to add to tea. Ginger relieves nasal problems, stress, depression, stomach problems and migraine headaches. Adding a few slices of ginger to your tea can provide these benefits.

3. Mint leaves
Fresh mint leaves applied in herbal tea will help improve your digestion. It gives strength to the body to fight against germs. Apart from this, it helps in reducing tension and headaches. It is not necessary to add more to the tea. It is enough to give a little two-one drops in tea.

4. Yellow

Turmeric works very well in improving the skin. And it can be drunk with tea. Apart from the skin, turmeric works as a beneficial ingredient for improving digestion and blood in the body. And when added to tea, it will not change the taste much. And the body can easily accept it as a beneficial element.

5. Basil leaves

Basil leaves can be used much like mint leaves. It is useful in improving your digestion when applied in herbal tea. It gives strength to the body to fight against germs. Apart from this, it helps in reducing tension and headaches.

6. Cayenne pepper

It is a type of red pepper that is beneficial for health. It increases blood circulation in the body, reduces stress and helps improve metabolism. Applying it in small amounts in your herbal tea can provide benefits.

7. Lavender oil

Lavender is a beautiful purple flower called lavender. Its oil has many beneficial properties. Infused in your tea, it will reduce stress, relieve your sleep problems and improve your nervous system. It works by adding a very small amount (one or two drops) to the tea.

The extraordinary qualities of ordinary peanuts

There is no pair of peanuts for leisure or chat. Groundnut is popular as 'timepass food' not only in Bangladesh but all over the world. Of all the types of nuts produced in the world, groundnut is the most widely used and popular. Apart from raw and roasted nuts, groundnut is also used in making butter, jam, chanachur, cakes, biscuits, curries, bhartas, oil etc.

Although the word 'China' is present in groundnut, it was first discovered in South America. There are traces of its cultivation even in ancient times. Many ancient vessels found in Lima, Peru, have images of almond trees painted on them. It is believed that eating almonds was common even during the time of the Inca civilization. Because, almond-shaped vessels have been found among the pottery of the Incas.

Peanuts were brought to Europe by the Spanish. Like tobacco leaves, nuts were also used as a medium of exchange. Later European traders took groundnuts to Africa. They gave groundnuts to the Africans in exchange for ivory and spices. Nuts eventually made their way to North America from Africa via African slaves.

 The practice of eating peanuts in the United States began before their Civil War. But then it was more common as food for domesticated animals. Some soldiers chose groundnuts as an alternative food when food was scarce during the war.

Later it gradually gained popularity among the soldiers. Shortly after the end of the Civil War, PT Barnum, the owner of a circus troupe, began selling roasted nuts during the circus, and roasted nuts became very popular. Many hawkers then turn to groundnut roasting as a new source of income.

Currently, China produces 41% of the total production of groundnuts in the world. That is probably why this nut is called groundnut.

English name of Chinese nut is Ground nut. Groundnut is the only nut that grows underground. Its scientific name is apios americana. However, groundnut is known as Peanut around the world.

It is named Peanut because it looks like a 'P' or a pea. It is also called 'Mankinat'. This name may be because the monkey community is particularly fond of this nut!

Many people may not care about groundnuts as they are easily available compared to other nuts. But groundnut is not less in any part in terms of food quality. Per 100 grams of raw groundnut contains –

Carbohydrates 60 grams Protein 53.3 grams Dietary energy 566 kcal Calcium 90 mg Iron 350 mg carotene 37 micrograms Vitamin B1 0.90 mg Vitamin B2 0.30 mg Roasting nuts reduces their carotene value. But all the other ingredients remain almost the same. Groundnut has many contributions to health. For example –

Peanut protein helps in body building and muscle building.
Its co-enzyme protects the heart from lack of oxygen.
Peanuts contain monounsaturated fats. It helps in controlling blood cholesterol.

It contains high levels of niacin which protects the body cells. Helps prevent age-related dementia diseases such as Alzheimer's. Keeps brain healthy and helps blood circulation.

Groundnut helps prevent colon cancer, breast cancer and heart disease.

It is rich in calcium, which helps in bone formation. Groundnuts are rich in iron, which helps in red blood cell function.

Vitamin E and carotene in groundnut keep skin and hair beautiful. Delays skin wrinkles.

<u>Important topic note please</u>

10 SIMPLE WAYS TO INCREASE STRENGTH IN THE BODY

Strengthening the body is very important for improving mental and physical health with proper dedication and leading a good lifestyle as well as a harmonious lifestyle. Here are some simple ways, which if used recently can help the body to increase energy:

1. Benefits of Adequate Diet:

Ensure completeness of food with proper amount of protein, vegetables, fruits and energy sources. For protein visit, you can start with animal feed (meat, chicken, egg), cow's milk, whey, fat-free milk etc. Vegetables, fruits and energy sources include pulses, green leafy vegetables, red salmon, vitamin C and more fruits.

2. Adequate water intake:

Water accelerates and is consumed in normal body functions. So take at least 8-10 glasses of water a day.

3. Set bedtimes and wake-ups:

Make sure to go to bed and wake up at set times. At least 7-8 hours of sleep should be taken every day. Observe for any type of air consumption.

4. Healthy break:

Instead of entertaining during the day, take a short rest break after class. It can help you increase energy and comprehension and list tension in mind]

5. Benefits of Exercise

----

and Sperm Increase: Make time for regular exercise. Maybe 30 minutes of moderate exercise.

6. Strong Mindset:

An important source of strength is mental state. Learn the flow and apply fluency. Think about the application of patience, intelligence and meditation.

7. Pranayama:

Chanting according to Nin and drawing the syllables with Ayam. It is good for improved respiration and strong body.

8. Healthy Mindset:

Maintain a healthy and balanced mindset. Apply intelligence to the state of mind test and keep in mind what you want to achieve.

9. Regular Massage:

Healthy massage is best when it has the correct circulation in the anatomy and blood circulation in the body.

10. Sure Rag Duruh:

Do Duruh regularly like safely and in half life. Wear soft and loose clothing.

Do daily breathing with this flow and ensure your full health with care. Comment: Please refer to the article completely with any advice as per your health.

<u>THESE ARE BONUS TIPS FROM ME</u>

Boosting energy is possible through regular exercise and a well-balanced nutritional diet. Here are two important points:

1. Serving of adequate amount of nutritious food: Food should be served in the right amount of energy-boosting elements such as protein, carbohydrates, fats, vitamins, and minerals. Your nutritious diet should include vegetables, fruits, complementary foods and protein sources such as meat, fish, milk.

2. Exertion and physical exercise: Energy development cannot be achieved when mental and physical activity is reduced. Exercising regularly and doing various physical exercises such as stretching, jogging, sitting, etc. develop strength in the body.

 These two points if followed properly will help increase body strength. Remember, a strong and healthy body is necessary to perform any task.

Designer and writer: Suvadra Rani Mondal

www.ingramcontent.com/pod-product-compliance
Lightning Source LLC
Chambersburg PA
CBHW070757250726

48662CB00004B/1849